A KEATS GOO[D HEALTH GUIDE]

HERBS FOR WOMEN'S HEALTH

Herbal help for the female cycle from PMS to menopause

Mary Bove, N.D. and
Linda Costarella, N.D.

Keats Publishing, Inc. New Canaan, Connecticut

Herbs for Women's Health is intended solely for informational and educational purposes, and not as medical advice. Please consult a medical or health professional if you have questions about your health.

HERBS FOR WOMEN'S HEALTH

Library of Congress Cataloging-in-Publication Data

Bove, Mary.
Herbs for Women's health / Mary Louise Bove, Linda Costarella.
p. cm.
Includes bibliographical references and index.
ISBN 0-87983-759-4
1. Generative organs, Female—Diseases—Treatment. 2. Herbs—Therapeutic use. 3. Self-care, Health. 4. Gynecology—Popular works. I. Costarella, Linda. II. Title.
RG129.H47B68 1997
618.1'06—DC21 96-52332
CIP

Printed in the United States of America

Published by Keats Publishing, Inc.
27 Pine Street (Box 876)
New Canaan, Connecticut 06840-0876

99 98 97 6 5 4 3 2 1

Contents

About the Authors

Mary Bove, N.D. is a naturopathic physician and midwife with a practice in family medicine and natural childbirth in Brattleboro, Vermont. A noted educator in herbal medicine, she is a member of the National Institute of Medical Herbalists in London and a former Chair of Botanical Medicine at Bastyr University. Dr. Bove is the author of *An Encyclopedia of Natural Healing for Children and Infants.* She lectures throughout the United States about botanical medicine, phytotherapy and naturopathic obstetrics.

Linda Costarella, N.D. is a naturopathic physician practicing in Saxton's River, Vermont. She earned her doctorate in naturopathic medicine from Bastyr University. Dr. Costarella is on the faculty of Vermont College of Norwich University and serves as Academic Dean at the North East College of Healing Arts and Science in Saxton's River, Vermont. Dr. Costarella has lectured widely and is published in the *Protocol Journal of Botanical Medicine.*

Introduction

From ancient times until the modern technological age, healthcare was mostly for, about and by women. The wonder of the reproductive cycle, the miracle of birth and the powerless mystery of death were the domains of women who watched over them. Before the dawn of patriarchy, women were the natural healers and guardians of the mysteries and stories of the people. Women looked to the earth from where life began and where the food for sustaining life was grown for help in healing the ill. And abundant help was there—in the form of plants which alleviated pain, cleared sores, stopped bleeding.

Plants have played a major role in health care for much of history. Healers used plants as part of the normal course of healthcare. Throughout the ages, from one generation to the next, the knowledge of plant medicines was passed from one person to another. Old medical texts feature the use of herbal therapies for illness. The Merck Manual, today's popular handbook of medical knowledge, was still listing herbal remedies as standard therapies in the early part of the 20th century.

After the advent of miracle drugs in the early part of this century, the use of plants as medicine began to wane. Medical schools began what was to become a colossal love affair with pharmaceutical therapy. Plants were used only to find the magic "active constituent" whose physiological activities could be proven by double-blind lab tests. Then that constituent could be synthesized in a laboratory, packaged into a pill, injection or liquid and promoted to physicians who were seeking quick-acting drugs to relieve symptoms. Knowledge of plant medicine faded into the blur of human history.

Women were no longer respected as natural healers as earth-based religions honoring nature and her power were replaced with patriarchal religions and plant-based healing was replaced with the worship of the scientific method. While the majority of individuals seeking healthcare continued to be women, often seeking help with problems having to do with reproductive health, the majority of physicians were male. Herbal remedies used for "women's problems" were denigrated as "old wives' tales," and became even further buried in the past.

This negativity lasted until late in this century. Today alternatives to the pharmaceutical approach are sought by at least a third of the U.S. population and there is renewed interest in herbal preparations for healing and preventing illness. Alternative medical schools train a corps of students that is approximately 66 percent female, and the role of women in health care has once again become very important. Every day the use of herbal therapies gains more and more respect.

Herbal preparations generally present few if any side effects. Many of the herbal combinations prescribed offer tonifying or balancing effects in the body. The underlying principle in the use of herbal remedies is that the body is already trying to heal itself. Our bodies attempt to maintain and restore homeostasis or balance to our physiological mechanisms whenever possible. On occasion, due to additional stress on the body or due to an exceptionally resistant causative agent, the body needs help. The more gentle and natural that help, the fewer side effects.

Thus, we offer this discussion of herbs that are useful in the treatment of women's health problems. We recommend considering the use of herbs before pharmaceuticals whenever possible. However, we strongly encourage all women seeking elimination of health problems to seek the help of a qualified herbal specialist or alternative healthcare provider if there is any question about the nature of the illness. We do not recommend self-diagnosis. This book is offered for information and educational purposes, but it is not intended for use without a medical assessment made by a qualified practitioner.

We have tried to make the instructions on the use of herbal therapies as straightforward as possible, and an appendix is offered to help obtain supplies for herbal preparations.

As stated earlier, women seek healthcare more often than men in our society. There have been many theories as to why this is the case. Certainly the complexity of the female reproductive cycle must account in part for this difference. Variations in the normal physiology of the cycle can account for a myriad of problems including painful periods, irregular periods, no periods, heavy periods, premenstrual discomfort, infertility, menopausal discomfort, breast tissue changes, ovarian growths, uterine growths and irritation and infections of the vagina (vaginitis). Due to the structure of the female urinary tract as compared to that of the male, women also generally have more frequent urinary tract infections (UTIs) than do men.

In this book, we will discuss many of the most common problems arising from disruptions of the normal female reproductive physiology and problems such as UTIs and vaginitis. We will also present a discussion of the herbal preparations which, over the years, have been found useful in dealing with these problems.

WHAT IS NOT IN THIS BOOK

There are many aspects of women's health which could not be covered in this small book. Some of those issues require an in-depth discussion of causes and treatments. For example, we have not discussed cancers of the breast, ovary or endometrium, sexual abuse, HIV-AIDS or sexually transmitted diseases.

However, the recommendations in this book regarding diet, nutrition and herbal therapeutics might prevent any illness involving the female reproductive system and would be helpful in dealing with the signs, symptoms and biochemical changes stemming from any of them. Once again, we strongly recommend that a thorough and complete diagnostic workup be done in order to assess the nature of any problems that exist.

The Structure of the Female Reproductive Organs

The Ovaries

The ovaries, often referred to as the "gonads" in women, are internal structures which are attached to the uterus near the fallopian tubes. They are attached to the uterus by a ligament known as the ovarian ligament. Each of the two ovaries normally found (one on each side of the pelvis) is approximately 3.5 × 2 × 1.5 cm. After menopause, the ovaries tend to get smaller and may measure only 2 × 1 × .5 cm.

Each ovary has several layers of tissue. Within one of these layers are tiny follicles which respond to hormonal changes and house the egg before ovulation. The ovaries produce two of the major hormones of the female reproductive cycle: these are estrogen and progesterone. The ovaries will secrete these hormones in response to messages from certain areas of the brain. The hormonal cycle of the human female is complex and there are many interrelationships. Some of these are covered in the next chapter.

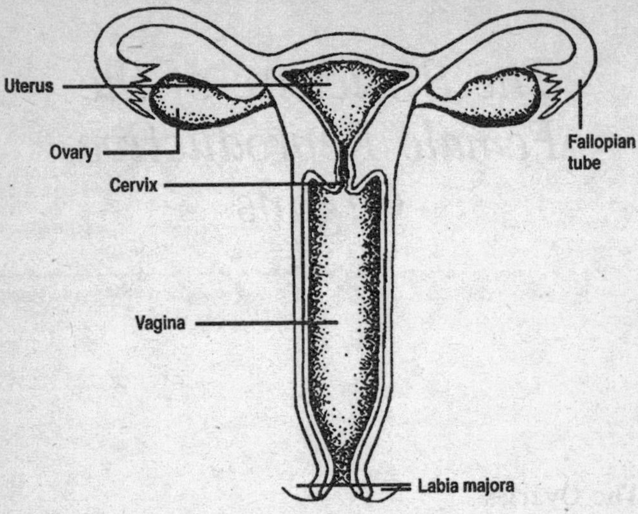

The Female Reproductive Organs

Every woman is born with all the eggs that she will ever have. These are the eggs that will develop under hormonal influence into mature eggs ready for fertilization.

The Uterus

The uterus lies between the rectum and the urinary bladder. It is usually approximately 3 × 5 × 7 cm in size. This organ is hollow, and its walls are composed of three layers. The outermost layer is known as the peritoneum and is the same structure that lines other organs in the abdominal cavity. The middle layer is known as the myometrium. This muscle is quite thick and smooth and is under the control of the autonomic nervous system; thus the movements of the uterus are not voluntary. The inner layer of the uterus is known as the endometrium. This is the layer that is rich in blood vessels. During the hormonal cycle, the endometrial lining enlarges in response to estrogen (as is discussed in the next chapter). Blood vessels in this layer eventually get deprived of blood, wither and eventually are shed as menstrual blood. If an egg is fertilized and enters the uterus, it will attach to the endometrium, and hormonal changes from that event will cause blood to continue to flow into the area so that the endometrium does not shed. It will, instead, be a source of enrichment and nourishment for the growing embryo.

The lower end of the uterus narrows to enter the vagina. The part of the uterus that extends into the vagina is known as the cervix.

The Cervix

The cervix is approximately 2.5 cm long. That portion of the uterus which extends into the vagina, the cervix has two openings—one at the uterine end called the *internal os* and one at the end that is visible in the vagina called the *external os*. The cells of the outside of the cervix are continually sloughed off into the vagina. A scraping of the cervix and vagina to obtain some of these cells is done in the procedure known as the Pap smear. Once placed on a slide, these cells are examined under microscope to be certain that they are normal.

Mucus is produced in the cervix and it changes with the hormonal changes of the normal reproductive cycle. This mucus can be examined in order to help determine where a woman is in her cycle and it can be used to aid in family planning by ensuring that measures are taken during the most fertile part of the cycle to avoid or to increase the chances for pregnancy. Fertility awareness is beyond the scope of this book. Also, while there are several common problems associated with the cervix, this book does not address them due to the complexity of the treatments.

The Vulva and The Vagina

The vulva is the external skin folding of the female genitals. It consists of the *labia majora* and the *labia minora,* the two surrounding "lips" of the opening of the vagina. The vagina is the internal canal that extends from the vulva to the cervix. The walls of tissue lining the vagina are mucous membranes which contain folds that enable the tissue to stretch during intercourse. There are normal stores of glucose (the body's major energy source) called glycogen in the vagina on which the many normal bacteria feed. This process maintains the vagina in an acid range, prohibiting the growth of many unfavorable bacteria and yeast. When that acidity is altered, infections of bacteria or yeast are more possible. Sperm need a less acidic environment in which to swim. Thus they will secrete a chemical to lessen the acidity in the vagina—a must for their survival.

The Breast

Female breasts consist of glandular tissue which is surrounded by protective fatty and connective supportive tissues. Called mammary glands, their glandular tissue develops initially before a baby girl is born and will mature under puberty's hormonal influences. The area around the nipple is known as the *areola.* Within the nipple there are milk ducts, sensory nerves and small involuntary muscles which contract under the influence of temperature and sexual stimulation.

Within each breast there are 15 to 20 lobes, each of which sends a duct to the nipple. The ducts join together to form larger openings. The lobes divide into 20 to 40 smaller lobules. Within the lobules are alveoli which secrete the milk to be sent through the ducts to the nipple. This process is under the control of the pituitary gland in the brain.

The Urinary Tract

The structure of the lower part of the female urinary tract can be the reason for frequent urinary tract problems including inflammation and infection. Since this is a common complaint in female health, it is included in this book.

The urinary tract includes the two kidneys which are situated posteriorly in the midback region. Each of these kidneys has a structure (the ureter) which connects to the urinary bladder located in the lower abdomen in front of the uterus. From the bladder, another tube extends down to just above the vagina. In women, this structure is much shorter than in men. It is also closer to the rectum, which may increase the likelihood of urinary tract infection from rectal bacteria. It is not unusual for women to mistake a vaginal infection for a urinary tract infection or vice versa due to the proximity of symptoms for each.

The Normal Female Reproductive Cycle

The Hypothalamus and Pituitary

The normal cycle in the human female involves a complex communication among several glands and organs. In the brain an area known as the hypothalamus, a master control center for many bodily functions, secretes gonadotropin-releasing hormone (GnRH). This hormone signals the pituitary gland, a tiny gland in the brain which is attached to the hypothalamus by way of the hypothalamic-pituitary axis, to secrete several hormones depending on the perceived needs of the body. In the case of the gonadotropin-releasing hormone from the hypothalamus, the pituitary will secrete follicle-stimulating hormone (FSH) and luteinizing hormone (LH). These hormones will in turn signal the production of estrogen and progesterone.

The Phases of the Cycle

The production and release of brain hormones basically divides the female endocrine cycle into three distinct phases. The first is known as the follicular or preovulatory phase. This phase begins on the very first day of the woman's bleeding and lasts approximately 14 days. During the beginning of that phase,

FSH secretion is increased. This hormone does exactly as its name indicates: it stimulates the development of follicles, a structure containing an egg and other cells in the ovary. Only one of these follicles will ovulate while the others will degenerate. During this time LH begins to rise slowly as well, and estrogen and progesterone are produced by the ovaries in constant low levels.

The ovulatory phase is a complex mechanism resulting in a surge of LH release by the pituitary. The egg is released from the follicle due to this LH surge. While estrogen production begins to increase slowly several days before the surge, it increases much more rapidly and peaks about a day before the LH surge. The FSH level begins to fall once the follicle has been developed. Also just before the LH surge, progesterone levels begin to increase significantly. Unlike estrogen, which peaks at the LH surge, progesterone continues to rise after the surge.

The postovulatory phase, also known as the luteal phase, is so named because of the *corpus luteum,* the supportive structure of the released egg. The production of progesterone becomes the task of the corpus luteum during this phase. Progesterone peaks on about the eighth day after the LH surge. At this time LH and FSH levels remain low only to begin the cycle over again by increased secretion when bleeding occurs. Hormones that mark the beginning or cessation of phases of the cycle have effects on other parts of the body besides the ovaries. Certainly the uterus responds dramatically to changes in hormone levels. Estrogen causes the lining of the uterus to thicken, engorging itself with a rich blood supply so that a fertilized egg can be implanted and nourished. Under the influence of progesterone, the lining of the uterus is encouraged to slough off, and bleeding occurs. Changes also occur in the vagina and the cervix (the "neck" of the uterus) due to fluctuations in these hormones. This includes the change in texture of cervical mucus, allowing a greater movement of sperm during the ovulatory phase.

Other areas of the body, outside the reproductive mechanisms, also respond to the hormones of the reproductive cycle. Breast tissue may enlarge and become sensitive due to the influence of estrogen. Body temperature is affected: there may be a rise in temperature just as the luteal phase begins or just before ovulation. Various studies have also shown increases in appetite, salt and water retention and even increases in the sensitivity of the five senses, such as more acute hearing or smell. Estrogen has been studied a great deal since the increased use of hormone replacement therapy, and the effects of estrogen on many body functions has been demonstrated again and again.

Menstruation

Menstruation, or the period of time in which bleeding normally occurs, begins approximately 28 days after the end of the last period and lasts approximately four to seven days, occurring technically in the pro-ovulatory cycle. As with the length of time of the three distinct phases, the number of days of bleeding can vary. The very first time a young girl experiences menstruation (menarche) may occur anytime from age 10 to age 16. Some girls begin before age 10 and some begin after age 16, but this is unusual. Periods will stop generally anywhere from age

40 to 55, the onset of menopause. We will discuss menopause as a separate chapter in more detail later.

The Adrenal Glands

The two adrenal glands are situated on top of the kidneys. These little glands have a major role in many bodily functions. They are responsible for helping to maintain mineral balance in the body as well as helping to control glucose levels, especially in times of stress. They also help adjust blood pressure when needed. The adrenal glands help when the body needs to shift metabolic processes towards rebuilding during and after times of stress. Steroid hormones are produced by the adrenal glands for this purpose. The adrenals also produce some estrogen and progesterone as well as the androgen hormones, which have a major role in helping to rebuild proteins degraded as a result of stress. Stress can include not only psychological distress but also physiological stressors such as illness, chronic allergies, toxic exposure, excess exercise or nutritional deficits due to starvation, malabsorption, maldigestion or parasitic infections.

The Liver

The liver also plays an important role in the metabolism of female hormones. The liver, in general, has the enormous task of detoxifying external substances which come into the body. What it also must do, however, is detoxify substances from within the body which might cause problems if allowed to build up. With the liver's help, these compounds are altered in such a way as to allow for their excretion by the body's complex elimination systems. The most appropriate example of this for purposes of this discussion is the liver's role in detoxifying estrogen metabolites.

As estrogen is broken down, it must go through the liver in order for the metabolic by-products to be made nontoxic and for them to be excreted from the body. The mechanisms the liver uses for this job are the same ones that are used to detoxify many other toxins or potential toxins in the body. This means that cigarette smoke, caffeine, alcohol, prescription drugs, the chemicals from auto exhaust and many other hormonal by-products go through this detoxification system in the liver. In addition, hormones taken in as prescriptions (oral contraceptive pills or hormone replacement therapy) are also detoxified here. Hormones may also be added to the liver's load from the foods that we eat such as red meat, cheese or chicken if the animals' feed contained hormones to make them grow larger. This may mean that the liver is very overworked, and may not be able to do its job properly. If this is the case, estrogen metabolites may remain in the body much longer than they should.

The effects of this overload will vary, depending on the woman's overall health and her genetic make up. Most often, hormonal regulation is altered in the body, creating disruptions of the normal reproductive cycle. Thus, irregular periods, heavy bleeding, or premenstrual symptoms may be experienced to one degree or another. Structural problems can also occur such as ovarian cysts, fibrocystic breasts or uterine fibroids. If the problem is serious enough, if there are other health problems in the woman, or if her family history so determines, breast cancer or uterine cancer may develop over time. Clear links between higher than normal estrogen metabolites and some forms of these diseases have been shown.

The Importance of Nutrients

There are many vitamins and minerals which are important in the production and elimination of hormones, the control of pain and inflammation in the body and the regulation and control of hormone release and utilization. It is important to assure that digestion is optimal and that the intestines are absorbing all that is needed in order to carry out these functions in a balanced way.

Vitamins which play an important role in the maintenance of a healthy reproductive system include the fat-soluble vitamins E and K and water-soluble vitamins B6, B5, folic acid, B12 and vitamin C. Minerals which are important for female health include calcium, magnesium, zinc and boron. Also important is maintenance of a balance of essential fatty acids in the body, for these will control the production of many of the active substances in the body that control pain and inflammation. Essential fatty acids are those which the body cannot produce on its own. Certain types of oils result in reduced inflammation and pain because of the compounds produced by them. Flaxseed oil, borage seed oil and evening primrose oil are three examples of oils which help control pain and inflammation in the body. A diet with adequate protein is also essential to provide the correct amino acids for the production of many important compounds.

Problems Which Can Occur

The complexities of the female hormonal cycle make it evident that, on occasion, there will be variations that create problems with the phases. If the communication among the organs and glands of the reproductive system falters, there may be too much estrogen or progesterone, creating a situation in which the episodes leading to the LH surge and the release of an egg do not occur in a timely fashion or at all. The resulting problems might be the absence of periods (amenorrhea), an excessively long cycle (oligomenorrhea), too frequent or too heavy periods (menorrhagia), bleeding between periods (metrorrhagia), painful periods (dysmenorrhea), failure to ovulate (anovulatory), inability to sustain a corpus luteum or other problems leading to infertility, discomfort before the period (premenstrual syndrome) or discomfort during the menopause. Other problems of hormonal imbalance may also exist such as fibrocystic breasts, uterine fibroids or ovarian cysts. We will discuss some of these in the following pages.

What About the Use of Oral Contraceptive Pills?

Regulating the hormone cycle with prescription hormone supplementation for purposes of birth control has been widely practiced and accepted for the past 35 years. Many women have gained a sense of freedom since these pills are exceptionally efficient in preventing pregnancy. Also, over the years, the formulas used in birth control pills have improved, lessening the side effects experienced by most women. Many women have used them successfully over the past 35 years feeling confident that they are entirely safe and often even essential for a couple wanting to avoid pregnancy.

We would like to caution, nonetheless, that the use of oral contraceptives is not for every woman. Even in women who seem to experience no obvious unpleasant side effects, the extra burden of the hormones (stronger and at times quite different from the form of hormone the body naturally makes) can increase liver and adrenal loads to the point that some problems eventually occur. The common scenario is that a woman takes these pills for a while in early marriage or before marriage, stops to have children, continues after bearing children and perhaps then goes on hormone replacement therapy as she goes through the menopausal changes. At the same time, many women experience uterine fibroids, ovarian cysts, fibrocystic breast disease and other problems which are not usually attributed to the pill. However, one should consider the possible links between the pill and these problems given the additional load on the liver. Genetics, lifestyle, and life's stresses all play a part in determining whether a woman develops problems caused by the pill.

Consideration should be given to natural family planning. Eliminating hormone supplementation prescribed as birth control would prevent a woman's chances of overloading the liver and developing the gynecological problems associated with that.

Problems with Menstruation

Absence of Periods

Amenorrhea is the term used to define the absence of menstruation. There are two types of amenorrhea: That which occurs when a young woman fails to start menstruating by the time she is in her midteens, and the cessation of periods once menarche has occurred for some reason other than menopause or pregnancy.

It is fairly uncommon for the first type of amenorrhea to occur. In order for a diagnosis of the cause of such a problem, the physician or other healthcare practitioner would need to have a thorough history from the patient including a family history. The physical examination is also an important tool in assessing the reasons for failure to menstruate. If periods have failed to come on by the age of 18, this type of evaluation should be undertaken. If the patient has not developed secondary female characteristics (growth of breasts, enlarged hips, pubic hair, etc.) by the age of 16, evaluation should occur at that time rather than waiting to age 18. Of course, anytime a problem is suspected, an evaluation including a history, physical examination and any laboratory tests which may be appropriate should be begun. The evaluation may include various tests including laboratory studies to indicate the levels of hormones present.

Cessation of periods is more common and may be the result of many variables. The first to consider, of course, is pregnancy or, depending on the age of the woman, menopause. These are the two most common causes of cessation of periods. If these causes are ruled out, an assessment should be done to ascertain whether the problem lies in the hormones being produced by the hypothalamus and pituitary or as a result of ovarian dysfunction. In addition, hormonal imbalances can occur as a result of stress, including both physiological (such as excess physical exercise) and psychological stress. In this case the adrenals work overtime to produce the necessary stress hormones, thereby depleting the ingredients needed for reproductive hormones.

Conventional Medical Treatments

Conventional treatment for amenorrhea depends on whether the cause relates to a structural or hormonal problem. On rare occasions the problem requires surgery to correct an anatomical problem. Usually, treatment involves the use of hormonal therapy. Estrogen and progesterone may be given to ensure that the patient goes through a normal reproductive cycle. Interference with the body's diversion of substances to other than reproductive hormones may also be attempted in order to get the body to begin making the appropriate female reproductive hormones.

Natural and Herbal Treatments

Diet

Eat a whole foods diet, low in animal fats and hydrogenated fats and high in raw vegetable oils, raw nuts and seeds and organic vegetables. Avoid coffee, other caffeinated drinks, chocolate, alcohol and refined carbohydrates. These foods stress the female reproductive system and leach out minerals and essential fatty acids. Include seaweed soups and salads in the diet to support the thyroid function. (See Dietary Sources of Phytoestrogen, page 76.)

Supplements

- B6 deficiency is associated with the absence of menstruation. Take 150 to 250 mg daily.
- Zinc is commonly associated with absence of menses, low immune function, stretch marks and poorly healing skin wounds. Take 15 to 30 mg daily.
- Evening primrose oil, black currant seed oil, or flaxseed oil can be helpful in providing the needed materials to build adequate hormones. Take 1,000 to 3,000 mg daily of any one of the above oils.

Exercise

Excessive exercise can lead to low body weight and loss of menses. Practice moderate, regular exercise balanced with a diet that has adequate calories for your weight and size.

Light

The use of full-spectrum lighting in your home or work space has a positive effect on the pituitary gland and can be very helpful in regulating the reproductive cycle. Getting out in the natural sunlight and moonlight regularly without sunglasses can also be helpful.

Herbal Treatments

It is important to create an herbal protocol which addresses the whole picture. Choose herbs to balance the hormonal cycle and encourage the body to produce adequate hormones. Include the phytoestrogen herbs such as alfalfa, red clover, licorice and black cohosh. Include vitex to regulate ovulation and pituitary function.

Also include reproductive tonic herbs to nourish, strengthen and regulate such as false unicorn root, motherwort, blue vervain, squaw vine and dong quai. I like to use these herbs in a tea or tincture over a period of three to six months. For good circulation to the pelvic area, which is a necessity for a healthy cycle, add a little rosemary, ginger or cinnamon to the hormone-balancing herbs. If stress is part of the overall picture include some calming and relaxing herbs such as lavender flowers, oat grass, chamomile or pasqueflower. Lastly, the liver should be supported with its work of breaking down hormones and toxins in the body. Herbs such as milk thistle seed, dandelion root, yellow dock or fennel seeds may be used for this.

Formula to Stimulate Menses

2 parts vitex
1 part alfalfa
1 part licorice root
1 part motherwort
1 part rosemary
1 part blue vervain

Steep 1 tsp. of the dried herb mixture in 1 cup boiling water for 10 minutes and strain. This mixture may be used as a tea: 1 cup 3 times a day; or as a tincture: take ½ to 1 tsp. 3 times a day.

IRREGULAR PERIODS

Oligomenorrhea is the term used for infrequent periods. Normally the three phases of the cycle occur within 21 to 35 days. Periods occurring longer than every 35 days may be the result of a problem which warrants investigation. It is likely that a hormonal irregularity exists that is suppressing the onset of menses. Since periods are continuing, the likelihood of a structural problem causing infrequent periods is remote. One should not rule out the possibility of pregnancy when periods seem to become irregular. It is not uncommon for a woman to bleed in her first trimester of pregnancy, and it is possible that she has mistaken this bleeding for a period. If the woman is of reproductive age and sexually active, this possibility should be considered.

If periods occur more frequently than every 21 days, the condition is called polymenorrhagia. Again, the likelihood is that there are hormonal imbalances creating the situation. Stress may be the cause of hormonal imbalance. As stated earlier, stress may initiate the production of hormones other than those necessary for normal female reproduction, in which case there may be a shortage of these hormones.

Tests to ascertain the levels of hormones in the blood may help to determine the cause of menstrual irregularities. Several types of tests exist, but perhaps the two most common are blood tests which can determine the levels of estrogen, progesterone, FSH and LH as of the day the test is performed, and a saliva test which is done on 11 different days during the cycle. This latter test can indicate a woman's progesterone and estrogen levels on the 11 representative days of her cycle. A chart of these levels, compared to a chart of normal hormone activity, may give a clear picture of whether hormonal irregularities are the cause of the infrequent periods. Usually this is the case. Of course, if a woman is taking oral contraceptive medication, there is the possibility that her periods are quite scant and therefore are perceived not as periods, but as some other irregularity such as midcycle bleeding; the more substantial flow periods may be perceived as periods that are far apart.

Other causes to consider in oligomenorrhea are the use of other drugs, whether prescribed or recreational. Some drugs used to treat psychosis, high blood pressure and some narcotics may have an effect on the normal cycle. Other causes to be considered are stress, weight loss, exercise and chronic disease. Again, these processes involve physiological changes which may account for hormonal irregularities. Cholesterol is a major building block for the production of steroid hormones, including the female reproductive hormones. Vitamins and minerals act as cofactors in the production and degradation of hormones. These can be deficient if there is a situation involving prolonged or acute stress or illness. As stated earlier, many of these nutrients will be selectively used for hormones and compounds that the body will use to reverse the effects of stress or illness. Exercise itself, when done in greater than moderate amounts, may stress the body, initiating the mechanisms addressed above.

Another consideration may be the health of the glands involved in the production of all of these hormones. Therefore, the health of the pituitary, hypothalamus, adrenal glands and ovaries should be examined. The ovaries may have growths on them which affect the types of hormones being produced by them. Since hormones from any gland act as chemical messengers to effect changes in cells in various parts of the body, and since glands communicate with each other exclusively through the production and secretion of hormones, it is evident that alterations in these chemicals may greatly alter normal hormonal regulation.

Conventional Medical Treatments

Conventional treatment involves the use of hormone replacement therapy, that is the use of estrogen and progesterone at certain parts of the cycle in order to balance the influence of these two hormones and establish more normal periods. Hormone replacement therapy often helps regulate periods by ensuring that the reproductive cycle functions as it ought to. However, the major shortcomings of this type of therapy are that the liver's load of hormonal checks and balances may be increased beyond its capacity. Moreover, synthetic hormone replacement does not address the underlying causes of hormonal dysregulation.

Natural and Herbal Treatments

Diet

Follow a whole-foods diet, low in animal fats and hydrogenated fats and high in raw vegetable oils, raw nuts and seeds and organic vegetables. Avoid coffee, other caffeinated drinks, chocolate, alcohol and refined carbohydrates. These foods stress the female reproductive system and leach out minerals and essential fatty acids. Include seaweed soups and salads in the diet to support the thyroid function.

Supplements

- B6 deficiency is associated with irregular menstrual cycles and premenstrual syndrome. Take 150 to 250 mg daily.
- Vitamin E can be very useful in regulation of the cycle; take 400 to 800 IU daily.
- Evening primrose oil, black currant oil or flaxseed oil can be helpful in providing the needed materials to build adequate hormones. Use 1,000 to 3,000 mg daily of any one of the above oils.

Exercise

Excessive exercise can lead to a lower body weight and loss of menses. Practice moderate, regular exercise balanced with a diet with adequate calories for your weight and size.

Light

The use of full-spectrum lighting in your home or work space has a positive effect on the pituitary gland and can be very helpful in regulating the reproductive cycle. Getting out in the natural sunlight and moonlight regularly without sunglasses can also be helpful.

Herbal Treatments

Vitex agnus-castus (also known as chaste tree) can be used as a tea, tincture or standardized extract in capsules. Vitex will restore the normal balance of estrogen and progesterone in the body, thus regulating ovulation and menstruation. Vitex should be taken continuously for 6 to 12 months.

Tincture: Take 40 drops of a 1:5 tincture each morning.
Standardized extract capsules: Take one 175 mg capsule each morning.

Choose herbs to balance the hormonal cycle, encourage the body to produce adequate hormones and tonify the reproductive system. Include the phytoestrogen herbs such as alfalfa, red clover, licorice, raspberry leaf, motherwort, lady's mantle, squaw vine and black cohosh.

There are many herbs that may be used to relieve stress and tension in the body and mind. Herbs such as oat grass, skullcap, lemonbalm and blue vervain are gentle nervous system tonics, while passionflower, valerian and kava kava are a little stronger in their action.

See Absence of Periods, page 18 for further herbs to consider.

HEAVY BLEEDING

Heavy bleeding is called *menorrhagia.* In some cases the term dysfunctional uterine bleeding (DUB) is used.

Miscarriage should be explored as a possible cause of the bleeding as should the use of hormones for birth control or hormone replacement or correction. Remember that the liver is trying desperately to keep up with the hormone load. If a woman takes hormones besides those that her body is producing, if she is also eating foods which are high in animal growth hormones, and/or if she has other heavy loads on her liver such as smoking, alcohol or caffeine, the liver will probably have an enormously difficult time carrying out its detoxification of hormones, resulting in a heavier than normal amount of circulating estrogen or progesterone.

Fibroid tumors on the uterus are the most common cause of heavy bleeding when there is a structural problem. The bleeding may be so excessive as to be considered a hemorrhage. There may be large clots, and the uterus may cramp and cause a great deal of pain. Other structural problems which may cause excessive bleeding include polyps or endometriosis. In many cases of heavy bleeding, the endometrium of the uterus has grown much thicker than it normally should. This often occurs after a period or several periods are missed. Hormonal imbalances have disturbed the normal shedding of the endometrial lining, but it continues to increase in size under the influence of estrogen. This is known as endometrial hyperplasia. Eventually the endometrial lining will slough off, but usually with a very heavy amount of blood, perhaps even hemorrhaging, and clots. Often this situation is also accompanied by uterine cramping.

In most cases, the liver is not functioning as well it should. Perhaps it is overloaded with toxins or it has been overloaded with hormones either from a pharmaceutical source or from the foods eaten. Often animals' feed contains hormones to make them grow larger or produce more milk. Stress may also play a major role, causing the adrenal glands to preempt the production of progesterone in favor of androgen hormones for rebuilding the body. This may cause a severe imbalance favoring too much estrogen, especially those parts of estrogen which should have been detoxified save for an overworked liver. When the liver is overworked, all bodily systems affected by estrogen will be more heavily challenged.

A hormone level evaluation would be an appropriate test at this point in order to help ascertain the cause of the excessive bleeding. A gynecological examination may bring the cause to light if a mass is felt. In this case, and often even if no mass is palpated, the patient may be sent for an ultrasound to determine whether there is a mass or whether the lining of the uterus has enlarged too much. At times, the healthcare practitioner may also consider the need for an endometrial biopsy which can aid in determining the cause of the excessive bleeding. The response of the uterus to estrogen is determined in such a study. Normally this would not be done if fibroids or polyps were found initially on ultrasound. In all cases, more serious causes of the bleeding, such as cancer, would be ruled out by testing and examination. This is especially true if bleeding occurs after menopause.

Conventional Medical Treatments

After a diagnosis has been made regarding the cause of the excess bleeding, the recommended course of action depends on the reason for the bleeding and on the size and nature of any structural problems which have been found. Hormonal therapy to correct imbalances in normal hormone regulation is usually the first consideration. If fibroids are found, hormones may be recommended to decrease their size, in the hope that by doing so the bleeding will decrease. If the fibroids are very large or numerous, hormones may be recommended for awhile until surgery can be safely performed to remove the fibroids. In some cases of DUB, a dilation and curettage (D&C) may be recommended. This procedure involves scraping the endometrium of the uterus. Often this procedure will stop the bleeding. If the underlying problems of diet and toxic exposure are not addressed, however, the problem may recur and in all likelihood a hysterectomy will later be recommended.

The major shortcomings of conventional medical treatments are that they do not address the underlying cause of the hormonal imbalances and they often present the body with additional stressors in the form of pharmaceutical hormones or surgery or both. Thus, the hormonal problems stemming from stressors or from poorly functioning glands are often not addressed at all. Instead, synthetic hormones are added to try to correct the problem by taking over the body's normal function, bypassing the glands that should be correcting themselves. These drugs can make the situation worse for two reasons. First, hormonal regulation in the body is usually carried out by a "checks and balances" system. If the body perceives that a hormone is produced in sufficient amounts, it will not continue producing that hormone. Thus, adding a hormone to the body, in effect, alters the production of natural hormones. Second, as stated earlier, the synthetic hormones (often of a different chemical nature than the hormones made by the body itself) need to be metabolized and detoxified by the liver. The additional load may make matters worse, especially if overload of the liver is the principal cause of the original problem.

If surgery is later required (and it often will be if the original problem has not been addressed), the stress on the body from surgery will further compromise the normal regulation of hormones. If the ovaries have been removed and the woman is much too young for menopause, hormone replacement will be ordered. A liver that could not handle the load of the woman's own hormones will certainly have difficulty dealing with the drugs. The excessive bleeding will have been corrected, but the liver load will only cause the problem to go elsewhere in the body.

Natural and Herbal Treatments

The herbal treatment approach would depend on the cause of the bleeding. See page 50 for the natural treatment of uterine fibroids. For heavy bleeding due to greater than normal endometrial growth, take the steps outlined below.

Diet

See The Antiestrogenic Diet, page 77.

Supplements

- Vitamin E can be very useful in the regulation of the menstrual flow; take 400 to 800 IU daily throughout the cycle. Increase by 400 IU two to three days prior to the onset of the menses and on the heavy days. If your bleeding is very severe vitamin E may be used at 800 IU every 4 hours while the bleeding is heavy. After several months of treatment the flow should be less heavy and the need for such high doses will lessen.
- Evening primrose oil, black currant seed oil or flaxseed oil can be helpful in providing the needed materials to build adequate hormones. Use 1,000 to 3,000 mg daily of any one of the above oils.
- Bioflavonoids can be supplemented to improve blood vessel integrity and circulation of blood flow to the area. Use in combination with vitamin C. The bioflavonoid dose is 200 to 500 mg 3 times a day.

Herbal Treatments

Take herbs that support and cleanse the liver such as dandelion root, burdock root, fennel seed, milk thistle seed, turmeric, artichoke or celandine. For example, drink an herbal decoction made from one or more of those herbs 2 to 3 times a day; take 2 milk thistle seed capsules 3 times a day; or take a tincture mixture of several of the above-named liver herbs at 1 tsp. 3 times a day for several months. Also include lemon juice, beets, artichokes and leafy green vegetables in your diet to aid the liver in its work.

Formula for Heavy Bleeding

Mix the following herbal tincture:

1 part yarrow flowers
1 part geranium root
1 part lady's mantle
2 parts shepherd's purse

Use ½ to 1 tsp. 3 to 4 times a day during the heavy days of the cycle.

Bleeding Between Periods

The term often used for bleeding between periods is *metrorrhagia.* The amount of bleeding will probably be a determining factor in finding the cause of this bleeding. It is not at all unusual for most women to experience this type of bleeding irregularity at some time in their menstrual life.

To determine the cause for metrorrhagia, it is important to know whether pregnancy may be the cause. It is not at all unlikely for bleeding to occur during the first trimester of pregnancy, and it may be perceived as a period or as bleeding between periods. Hormone pills such as the oral contraceptive pill may also cause bleeding at an abnormal time or in abnormal amounts. Another contraceptive device which may initiate irregular bleeding episodes is the intrauterine device (the IUD). At times bleeding may occur normally at ovulation. In this case, there may be a small amount of blood evident at the same time the egg is released, and the reason may be obvious because of its regularity during the menstrual cycle.

If none of the above is found to be the cause of bleeding between periods, other possibilities should be considered including polyps, endometriosis, problems with the cervix such as irregular cell growth (dysplasia), infection or even fibroids. Again, hormonal regulation is critical for a normal cycle. Therefore, an evaluation of hormone levels and metabolism are another avenue to pursue. Physical examination and ultrasound, Pap smear, and possibly biopsy are also important evaluation tools for determining why there is bleeding between periods.

Conventional Medical Treatments

The course of action for metrorrhagia depends on the findings from any tests or examinations performed. They may involve the removal of polyps, adjustment or initiation of oral contraceptive pills, removal or adjustment of an IUD, procedures to correct abnormal cervical cell areas, etc.

Natural and Herbal Treatments

Diet

Eat a whole foods diet, low in animal fats and

hydrogenated fats and high in raw vegetable oils, raw nuts and seeds and organic vegetables. Avoid coffee, other caffeinated drinks, chocolate, alcohol and refined carbohydrates. These foods stress the female reproductive system and leach out minerals and essential fatty acids. Include seaweed soups and salads in the diet to support the thyroid function.

Supplements

- B6 deficiency is associated with irregular menstrual cycles and premenstrual syndrome. Take 150 to 250 mg daily.
- Vitamin E can be very useful in regulation of the cycle; take 400 to 800 IU daily.
- Evening primrose oil, black currant seed oil or flaxseed oil can all be helpful in providing the needed materials to build adequate hormones. Take 1,000 to 3,000 mg daily of any one of the above oils.

Light

The use of full-spectrum lighting in your home or work space has a positive effect on the pituitary gland and can be very helpful in regulating the reproductive cycle. Getting out in the natural sunlight and moonlight regularly without sunglasses can also be helpful.

Herbal Treatments

Vitex should be used as a tea, tincture or standardized extract in capsules. Vitex restores the normal balance of estrogen and progesterone in the body, regulating ovulation and menstruation. Vitex should be taken continuously for 6 to 12 months.

Tincture: Take 40 drops of a 1:5 tincture each morning.

Standardized extract capsules: Take one 175 mg capsule each morning.

Choose herbs to balance the hormonal cycle, encourage the body to produce adequate hormones and tonify the reproductive system. Include the phytoestrogen herbs such as alfalfa, red clover, licorice, raspberry leaf, motherwort, lady's mantle, squaw vine, wild yam, blue cohosh and black cohosh. For good circulation to the pelvic area, which is a necessity for a healthy cycle, add a little rosemary, ginger or cinnamon to your hormone balancing herbs.

Herbal Formula for Bleeding Between Menses

Blend the following herbs as a tea or a tincture:

1 part wild yam
2 parts vitex
1 part blue cohosh root
1 part false unicorn root
2 parts raspberry leaf
1 part cinnamon bark

As a tea, you might find this somewhat unpleasant tasting. If you can tolerate it, drink 2 to 3 cups daily for 3 cycles. If you prefer, take it as a tincture, ½ to 1 tsp. 2 or 3 times a day for 3 cycles.

PAINFUL PERIODS

The term for painful periods is *dysmenorrhea.* In the past, it was thought that women complained unnecessarily of menstrual pain. Some were felt to be hypochondriacs or unable to tolerate normal pain. Now there is recognition that painful periods can be a serious and debilitating condition. Pain can be extremely severe, preventing women from going about the normal routine of life. Women have had to leave work or school, lie down for a day or more at a time and often find little relief from painkillers. The pain is in the lower abdomen and may be accompanied by pain in the lower back as well. At times there will be changes in bowel movement associated with the pain. It is not uncommon for constipation to accompany the early pain and diarrhea to accompany the onset of the period or the relief of pain.

In some cases the cause of the pain may be a structural problem such as uterine fibroids or endometrial hyperplasia. Another common cause of painful periods is endometriosis. In these cases, the structural problems themselves may be causing the pain.

In cases where there is no obvious structural problem, the pain may be the result of abnormal prostaglandin production. Prostaglandins control many body mechanisms including those having to do with pain and inflammation. Prostaglandins are active substances produced in the body when the need arises because of mechanisms that are not yet entirely understood. Fatty acids biochemically break down into several different prostaglandins, as stated earlier. Some of these increase the sensation of pain in the brain and are responsible for initiating the body's inflammatory response to injury. Inflammation will result in pain and swelling in the area of the body affected. Others moderate those effects by lowering pain and curtailing the inflammatory process.

The kinds of fatty acids consumed in the diet generally determine which kinds of prostaglandins will predominate when the need for them arises. Generally, fatty acids derived from animal fats and other saturated fats increase the production of pain-producing prostaglandins. Fats that have fewer pain-producing prostaglandins are less saturated fats such as evening primrose oil, borage seed oil, flaxseed oil, olive oil and fish oils.

Hormone changes may also be responsible for the body's release of pain-producing prostaglandins, but more research is needed in this area. However, balance of hormones is always the goal in order to prevent any irregularity in the menstrual cycle.

Conventional Medical Treatment

Conventional approaches to painful periods would be similar to that for other problems related to periods. The first thing would be to rule out any structural problems that may be causing the pain. Again, these would include fibroids, endometriosis, endometrial hyperplasia, etc.

In those cases where there is no obvious cause for the pain, and in all other cases as well, pain management would be the treatment of choice. Some medications used are those that alter prostaglandin production or are prostaglandin inhibitors. These are the well-known nonsteroidal anti-inflammatories (NSAIDs) which can be acquired without a prescription in most cases. Stronger doses usually require prescription. Other drugs that have been used in the treatment of painful menstruation include narcotics, antispasmodic medications and minor tranquilizers. At times oral contraceptives are used which have helped some women, presumably by altering prostaglandin regulation.

Natural and Herbal Treatments

Diet

Eat a whole foods diet, low in animal fats and hydrogenated fats and high in raw vegetable oils, raw nuts and seeds, and organic vegetables. Avoid coffee, other caffeinated drinks, chocolate, alcohol, and refined carbohydrates. These foods stress the female reproductive system and leach out minerals and essential fatty acids. Include seaweed soups and salads in the diet to support the thyroid function. Include whole grains, legumes, and fresh organic fruits and vegetables to provide plenty of fiber to keep the stools regulated as constipation will add to pelvic congestion and make cramps worse. See the Antiestrogenic Diet, page 77.

Herbal Treatments

Black Cohosh is an excellent antispasmodic for menstrual cramps and general pelvic discomfort. Use 1 cup of decoction made from the dry root or ½ tsp. tincture 3 times a day.

Jamaican Dogwood capsules or tincture will also relax the cramping and ease discomfort. Use ½ tsp. of the tincture 3 to 4 times a day or 2 100 mg capsules 3 times a day.

Crampbark (Highbush Cranberry) may be used as a tea or a tincture to ease menstrual cramps. It relaxes the smooth muscle of the uterus and decreases spasm of the cervical neck. Use a tea made from 1 Tbsp. of the dry herb to 8 oz. of water, simmer 10 minutes covered and drink 3 to 4 times a day or as needed. If using the tincture, use 1 to 2 tsp. per dose 3 to 4 times a day or as needed.

Black Haw acts very much like crampbark in relaxing the uterus. I often mix the two tinctures together and use them as described above.

Remedy for Menstrual Cramps

2 parts crampbark
1 part black haw
1 part raspberry leaf
1 part catnip
½ part ginger

This can be mixed as a tincture or a tea. If making a tea with the mix, use 2 tsp. herbal mix to 8 oz. of boiling water, steep 10 minutes and drink warm. If using the tincture, use ½ to 1 tsp. 3 to 4 times a day with a little warm water.

Relaxing Belly Oil

This oil may be rubbed over the pelvic area to relieve cramping, to decongest and to relax the area. Combine the following in a 4-ounce amber glass bottle:

3 oz. castor oil
10 drops each of rosemary, lavender and basil essential oils
½ oz. cayenne oil

Shake well and apply to abdomen for cramps. Cover with a towel and a hot water bottle or heating pad.

Evening primrose oil contains large amounts of gamma-linolenic acid (GLA) which will correct poor essential fatty acid metabolism and reduce breast tenderness by increasing anti-inflammatory prostaglandin production. Take 2,000 to 4,000 mg daily with meals.

Liver herbs. Using herbal medicines such as dandelion root, fenugreek seed, milk thistle and yellow dock to support the liver's job of breaking down hormones and processing waste products will help to decrease pelvic congestion and inflammation. Add to these herbs such as ginger, rosemary and prickly ash, which increase blood flow to the pelvic organs, and pelvic drainers such as horsetail, nettles, squaw vine and corn silk to move fluid from the area.

Liver Support Formula

2 parts dandelion root
1 part fenugreek seed
1 part squaw vine
1 part rosemary
1 part nettle

Mix together and use as a tincture. Take one tsp. 3 times a day starting 5 to 7 days before the menses is expected. Drink a tea for the rest of the cycle made from equal parts of fennel, fenugreek and milk thistle seeds. Use 1 Tbsp. to 8 oz. of water; simmer covered 5 minutes, strain and drink.

Premenstrual Syndrome (PMS)

Discomfort associated with the onset of the menstrual period is often referred to as premenstrual syndrome or PMS. At times painful periods have been called PMS, but it is generally a different mechanism that causes this syndrome.

Many women experience some sorts of changes prior to the advent of their periods. These changes may include increased fluid retention, increased sensitivity to emotional stimuli, lower back or abdominal pain, sleepiness, sleeplessness, increased or decreased hunger, cravings for certain foods (most notably chocolate or starchy foods), constipation, clumsiness, increased or decreased energy and depression or anxiety. Some women also experience headaches, tenderness in the breasts, acne or increased herpes outbreaks. Though there are a myriad of jokes about PMS, the problem can be very serious for some women, disrupting their daily life. Relationships can also be adversely affected by PMS. Women have blamed themselves for many years for any conflict that arises from PMS, assuming that they have simply been unable to handle the normal hormonal cycle. "Raging hormones" has been the expression used to describe any emotionality associated with women, and this expression has been also used to justify the exclusion of women from certain jobs. Fortunately that is changing, albeit slowly. Women are able to seek help for premenstrual symptoms without feeling as though they are hypochondriacs.

PMS can be classified into four types depending on the symptoms experienced.

1. The most common type usually involves feelings of anxiety, irritability and nervous tension as well as cravings for sweets and carbohydrates. Generally, the cause of this type of PMS is thought to be high levels of estrogen and low levels of progesterone in the body.
2. Symptoms of edema (swelling), bloating in the abdomen, pain in the breasts and weight gain are the hallmarks of this type of PMS. The underlying cause is thought to be retention of salt and water in the body due to imbalances in hormones other than reproductive hormones, perhaps caused in part by the interaction of the two.
3. In this case the symptoms are increased appetite, cravings for sweets, palpitations of the

heart, fatigue, fainting, headache and mood swings. These symptoms are thought to be caused by low levels of magnesium in red blood cells and by alterations in the body's regulation of blood sugar.

4. The least common of all four, this type of PMS may cause a woman the most problems. The symptoms are depression, sleep disturbances, lack of coordination, confusion and loss of concentration. Its cause is thought to be low levels of estrogen in the blood along with high progesterone levels. Often there are also elevated androgens secreted by the adrenal glands, which may cause acne as well.

It is important to note that, while this system of classifying PMS symptoms and causes is helpful as a whole in identifying a woman's individual needs in therapy, most women experience symptoms from more than one specific category or type. Thus there are women who experience water retention and headaches and irritability and depression. Each woman's symptoms must be examined not only in light of the hormonal and obvious physiological causes, but also in light of her own lifestyle and diet. Any medications and supplements taken need to be considered in the assessment as well as the woman's intake of caffeine and other substances, which have profound physiological effects in the body.

Conventional Medical Treatment

Therapy for PMS often includes hormone replacement for regulation of normal hormonal metabolism; generally synthetic progesterone is supplemented since the most common type of PMS involves a probable estrogen excess in relationship to progesterone. Diuretics may also be used to alter mineral content and water content in the tissue, relieving swelling and abdominal bloating in some cases. Even more complex pharmaceutical interventions can be employed in some cases, using tranquilizers and lithium to control anxiety and depression. Once again, these measures ignore the cause of the problems in favor of symptomatic relief. If the problem is in the liver, the use of pharmaceutical hormones and other drugs will only make matters worse over time. Diuretics often disrupt the normal workings of the kidney in regulating fluid levels in the body. A more natural approach would leave the kidneys functioning normally.

Natural and Herbal Treatments

Proper hormone regulation, optimal liver function and natural relief of symptoms are the key to a natural approach to dealing with PMS.

Diet

Eat a whole foods diet, low in animal fats and hydrogenated fats and high in raw vegetable oils, raw nuts and seeds, and organic vegetables. Avoid coffee, other caffeinated drinks, chocolate, alcohol and refined carbohydrates. These foods stress the female reproductive system and leach out minerals and essential fatty acids. Include seaweed soups and salads in the diet to support the thyroid function. Include whole grains, legumes and fresh organic fruits and vegetables to provide plenty of fiber to keep the stools regular as constipation will add to pelvic congestion, bloating and cramps. Avoid refined sugars and carbohydrates as they lead to reactive low blood sugar and promote cravings for sweets. If you have water retention as part of your PMS picture, avoid excessive salt use; processed, refined foods are often high in sodium. See the Antiestrogenic Diet, page 77.

Exercise

Regular exercise such as walking, swimming, dancing, aerobics or biking for 20 to 60 minutes a day can greatly reduce the severity of PMS. Meditative exercise, such as tai chi or yoga, can also be beneficial in relieving stress, tension and anxiety.

Supplements

- Evening primrose, borage or flaxseed oil, 1,000 to 3,000 mg daily.
- Vitamin B6, 100 to 300 mg daily.
- Vitamin E, 400 to 800 IU daily.
- Magnesium glycinate, 500 to 1,000 mg daily.

Herbal Treatments

The use of herbs in PMS should again focus on relieving the liver of its toxic load and regulating hormones. Some relief from symptoms may also be obtained.

Herbs useful for the liver include milk thistle, dandelion root, burdock, turmeric, celandine and artichoke. Herbs which help relieve the congestion in the pelvic area and fluid retention include dandelion leaf, horsetail and parsley.

Herbs to help with nervous tension include passionflower, valerian, oatgrass, lemonbalm and skullcap. The use of calcium and magnesium may also help to control nervous tension.

To regulate the hormonal cycle, helpful herbs include vitex, wild yam, licorice, alfalfa, and black cohosh.

These herbs can be taken in a tea or in tincture form.

PMS Formula

1 part dandelion root and leaf
1 part milk thistle
1 part vitex
1 part black cohosh
1 part wild yam

As a tea, steep 1 tsp. of the herbal combination in 1 cup of boiling water for 10 minutes and drink 3 times a day. If a tincture is used, take ½ tsp. 3 to 4 times a day.

Abnormal Growths of the Female Reproductive System

Ovarian Cysts

The most common type of ovarian cyst is the *follicular cyst* which is formed during that part of the hormonal cycle when the follicles are being formed. These cysts may cause only slight discomfort, a heaviness in the pelvic region of the abdomen. They may also cause irregular periods because of the unusually high amount of estrogen in the cyst. Rarely, this type of cyst may burst, causing a great deal more pain and possibly requiring medical attention.

A less common type of cyst is the *lutein cyst* which occurs during the formation of the corpus luteum in the hormonal cycle. It can cause irregular periods, and there is often a feeling of dull pain in the pelvis where the ovary is. If this cyst ruptures, medical attention should also be sought.

Cysts generally occur because of a hormonal problem resulting in the follicles or corpus luteum forming incorrectly. Once again, the regulation of hormones is critical in avoiding this phenomenon.

Conventional Medical Treatments

Unless the cyst ruptures or causes severe symptoms, the course of action is usually to wait until it resolves on its own. If the cyst persists and is causing great discomfort, it may be examined by laparoscope (a procedure in which the abdominal contents are viewed by inserting a fiberoptic scope through small incisions in the abdomen) to rule out more serious causes of the symptoms. Surgery may be required to remove the cysts (and usually the ovary) if there is no resolution.

Natural and Herbal Treatments

Diet

See The Antiestrogenic Diet, page 77. It is extremely important to avoid estrogen-aggravating foods and xenoestrogens in food sources. Estrogen stimulates the ovarian tissue and follicle growth. Include high fiber foods (whole grains, vegetables, fruits) in your diet as they stimulate the excretion of estrogen from the body. Caffeine and chocolate are particularly harmful at this time.

Supplements

- Evening primrose oil, 1,000 mg 2 or 3 times a day with meals.
- Beta-carotene, 75,000 to 150,000 IU daily.
- Vitamine E, 400 IU daily with a meal.
- A good quality, balanced multivitamin and mineral formula will provide extra antioxidant nutrients to aid the body in healing.

Herbal Treatments

General treatment goals would include balancing the hormones, decreasing exogenous estrogens, supporting liver function, decreasing inflammation in the pelvic area, promoting lymphatic drainage and aiding in the removal of toxins and waste from the body.

Choose herbs to balance the hormonal cycle, encourage the body to produce adequate hormones and tonify the reproductive system. Include phytoestrogen herbs such as alfalfa, red clover, licorice, motherwort and black cohosh and tonics like blue cohosh, false unicorn root, raspberry leaf, lady's mantle or blue vervain. Use these herbs for 3 to 6 cycles.

If you experience midcycle pain use antispasmodic and relaxant herbs to relieve the discomfort, along with heat to the area. Drink a cup of hot tea or take ½ tsp. of tincture of crampbark, valerian, passionflower or catnip. Mix with a little ginger or cinnamon to bring extra warmth to the area.

Working with herbs to support and cleanse the liver such as dandelion root, burdock root, fennel seed, milk thistle seed, turmeric, artichoke and celandine will aid the body in removing toxins, hormones and waste. This can be done by drinking an herbal decoction of several of these herbs 2 to 3 times a day; by taking 2 milk thistle seed capsules 3 times a day; or by taking a tincture mixture of several of these herbs at 1 teaspoon 3 times a day for several months. Also include lemon juice, beets, artichokes and leafy green vegetables in your diet to aid the liver in its work.

Liver and Lymphatic Tincture

2 parts milk thistle seed
2 parts dandelion root

1 part burdock root
1 part red root
2 parts cleavers

Take ½ to 1 tsp. 3 times a day for several weeks.

Castor oil packs. A pack can be placed over the ovary area for an hour several times a week. The castor oil helps to decongest the pelvic cavity, improve circulation of lymph and blood and aid immune function. Do not use the castor oil pack while menstruating. See page 79 for instructions.

Uterine Fibroids

The uterine fibroid is a benign tumor which grows either in the uterus or on the outside wall of the uterus. It is an overgrowth of the smooth muscle of the uterus. Although benign in 99.99 percent of the cases, a uterine fibroid can often cause considerable discomfort and irregular or heavy periods. At times, the bleeding may be so heavy that the woman suffers from anemia and may even need a blood transfusion. This level of severity is quite unusual, however. The woman may experience a feeling of heaviness in her pelvic area.

Ultrasound is often used to diagnose the problem.

Conventional Medical Treatments

These treatments usually consist of trying to keep on top of the symptoms. Thus, the doctor might prescribe iron for anemia, painkillers for pain and perhaps hormones to try to shrink the size of the fibroids. This last approach might even be used prior to a scheduled surgical procedure to remove the fibroids or the entire uterus, if that is deemed necessary due to the size or nature of the fibroids. Hysterectomy is a very common treatment for fibroids.

Natural and Herbal Treatments

Diet

Avoid caffeine in the forms of chocolate, coffee, black tea and colas. Reduce animal fats in the diet, particularly red meats and milk products. Avoid saturated oils and margarine. Use raw, cold-pressed vegetable oils such as olive, sesame or sunflower.

Include soy products in the diet regularly such as soy flour, miso, tempeh, soymilk and tofu. Eat whole grains and complex carbohydrates, limiting refined flours and sugar. Be sure the diet has adequate fresh organic fruits and vegetables.

See the Antiestrogenic Diet, page 77.

Supplements

Evening primrose oil contains large amounts of gamma-linolenic acid (GLA) which corrects poor essential fatty acid metabolism and reduces pelvic pain and inflammation by increasing anti-inflammatory prostaglandin production. Take 2,000 to 4,000 mg daily with meals.

Antioxidants such as vitamins C and E, beta-carotene and selenium help to reduce inflammation by stopping free radical activity which can damage cells, change cell structure and set off the inflammatory process.

- Vitamin C, 5 to 10 grams in divided doses daily (use buffered if digestion is sensitive).
- Vitamin E, 400 to 800 IU daily.
- Beta-carotene, 50,000 to 150,000 IU daily.
- Selenium, 200 mcg daily.

Herbal Preparations

Chaparral tea should be used only as a tea and not taken in other types of preparations such as capsules. Add ½ cup of dried chaparral to 2 quarts of cold water; simmer covered on low heat until half of the liquid is gone. Drink ¼ cup daily. Store tea in the refrigerator.

Vitex can be used as a tea, tincture or standardized extract in capsules. Vitex restores the normal balance of estrogen and progesterone in the body and reduces prolactin production in the second half of the cycle known as the luteal phase. Vitex should be taken continuously for 3 to 6 months.

Tincture: Use 40 drops of the 1:5 tincture each morning.

Standardized extract capsules: Use one 175 mg capsule each morning.

Herbal Formula for Fibroids

This formula helps to reduce pelvic congestion, improve liver function and increase pelvic circulation.

2 parts dandelion root
2 parts milk thistle seed
1 part squaw vine
1 part prickly ash
1 part false unicorn root
1 part yarrow flowers

1 part ginger root

Use as a tincture. Take ½ tsp. 3 times a day for several months.

Lavender and Yarrow Flower Sitz Bath

Make a strong infusion of lavender and yarrow flowers in equal amounts. Use 3 Tbsp. flower mix to 1 quart water. Steep 10 to 15 minutes and strain into a shallow-filled bath tub. Sit with only the pelvis covered with water for 20 minutes several times a week. Rinse pelvic area with cold water before drying.

Castor Oil Packs

A pack can be placed over the uterine area for an hour several times a week. The castor oil helps to decongest the pelvic cavity and improve circulation of lymph and blood. Do not use the castor oil pack while menstruating. See page 79 for instructions.

Formula for Heavy Bleeding

Mix the following herbal tincture:

1 part yarrow leaves
1 part geranium root
1 part lady's mantle
2 parts shepherd's purse

Use ½ to 1 tsp. 3 to 4 times a day during the heavy days of the cycle.

Endometroisis

Endometriosis is a painful chronic disease in which endometrial tissue grows outside of the uterus in the pelvic cavity. The ovaries, utero-sacral ligaments and the fallopian tubes are most commonly affected and sometimes the bladder or colon. The main theory for why endometriosis develops is that a retrograde spill flushes menstrual tissue back up the fallopian tubes and into the pelvic cavity thus carrying with it endometrial tissue. This tissue begins to grow, responding each month to the ovarian hormones, particularly estrogens. Treatment goals include reduction of circulating estrogens and balancing of the ovarian hormones. Common complaints associated with endometriosis include pelvic pain, painful periods, pain with intercourse, pelvic mass and infertility. Menstrual irregularities such as irregular cycles, heavy menses, premenstrual spotting and bleeding with ovulation may also be present. Diagnosis of the disease may be made only by visualizing the lesion. Most commonly this is done by laparoscopy.

Conventional Medical Treatments

Conventional treatments for endometriosis include hormone therapy to stop ovulation, pain medications and conservative laser surgery.

Natural and Herbal Treatments

Treatment of this condition naturally requires a holistic approach focusing on the underlying chronic imbalances as well as relieving symptoms during acute episodes of pain and discomfort. Long-term goals include improving and normalizing immune function, improving liver function and balancing hormone levels, particularly estrogens. Treatments need to be used for at least three months and commonly for 12 to 18 months.

Successful treatment of this condition requires many lifestyle changes. Eating a diet which is high in phytoestrogen foods and low in xenoestrogens for several months to a year will help to decrease the estrogen loads in the body. (See Antiestrogen Diet, p. 77) Drinking herbal teas will aid the liver in its detoxification processes.

Detox Tea

Mix several of the following herbs in equal proportions:

- Dandelion root
- Burdock root
- Fennel seed
- Fenugreek seed
- Milk thistle seed
- Yellow dock root

Prepare a decoction of the mixture and drink 1 cup warm each morning for several months.

Supplements

The use of supplements to decrease inflammation and free radical damage helps to lessen the immune system's work and enable the body to regulate itself. The regular use of essential fatty acids such as flaxseed oil or evening primrose oil is recommended. Take 1,000 mg 3 times a day with meals. Antioxidant vitamins and minerals provide extra support for the body. These may be supplemented in a multiple antioxidant formula or individually.

- Vitamin C, 5 to 10 grams daily; use buffered if your digestion is sensitive.
- Vitamin E, 400 to 800 IU daily.

- Beta-carotene, 50,000 to 150,000 daily.
- Selenium, 400 mcg daily.

Herbs

Vitex acts to regulate the hormonal cycle in the body by stimulating the pituitary gland to produce more luteinizing hormone (LH). This increases the production of progesterone in the second half of the menstrual cycle, which aids in checking the estrogens and creating a normal balance of estrogen and progesterone. Use 40 drops of the tincture or 2 capsules first thing in the morning for 6 to 18 months.

Licorice, alfalfa, red clover, black cohosh and dong quai are valuable for their phytoestrogen action upon the estrogen receptors. See Herbs Containing Phytoestrogens, page 76.

Ginger, rosemary or cinnamon used in tea formulas or as a hot tea on their own will help to increase pelvic circulation and drainage of pelvic waste. If taking an herbal tincture, add ¼ teaspoon of ginger tincture to every oz. of tincture for its medicinal action as well as its pleasant flavor.

Herbs for pelvic pain. See page 39.
Herbs for heavy bleeding. See page 31.

Topical treatments

Castor Oil Pack. Use 30 to 60 minutes several times a week except during menstruation. See Castor Oil Pack, p. 79.

Hot-Cold Sitz Bath (see p. 80).

Fibrocystic Breast Disease

In reviewing the anatomy of the breast, you will recall that the breast consists of fatty tissue, glandular tissue and connective tissue. These tissues can grow larger than normal and/or can become slightly hard. The lumps that are produced as a result of hormonal influences may be very tender and may change with the ebb and flow of the hormonal cycle. Generally breast lumps that change this way are benign. This is more likely if the lumps are movable when palpated and if they are tender. The pain can be severe at times; usually, however, fibrocystic breasts are only mildly tender.

Conventional Medical Treatments

Hormone treatment is sometimes prescribed, though not commonly. Generally the patient is given mild pain killers or diuretics. Mammograms may be prescribed to rule out cancer.

Natural and Herbal Treatments

Diet

- Avoid caffeine in the forms of chocolate, coffee, black tea and colas.
- Reduce animal fats in the diet, particularly red meats and milk products.
- Avoid saturated oils and margarine. Instead use raw, cold-pressed vegetable oils such as olive, sesame or sunflower.

- Include soy products in the diet regularly such as soy flour, soymilk and tofu.
- Eat whole grains and complex carbohydrates, limiting refined flours and sugar.
- Be sure the diet has adequate fresh, organic fruits and vegetables.
- See Antiestrogenic Diet, page 77.

Supplements

Evening primrose oil contains large amounts of gamma-linolenic acid (GLA) which acts to correct poor essential fatty acid metabolism and reduces breast tenderness by increasing anti-inflammatory prostaglandin production. Use 2,000 to 4,000 mg daily with meals.

Vitamin E can be helpful in reducing breast tenderness and cysts of the breast. It also helps to reduce inflammation of the breast tissue and quench free radicals in the body. Take 400 to 800 IU daily.

Herbal Preparations

Vitex can be used as a tea, tincture or standardized extract in capsules. Vitex acts to restore the normal balance of estrogen and progesterone in the body and reduces prolactin production in the second half of the cycle known as the luteal phase. Vitex should be taken continuously for 3 to 6 months.

Tea: Use one Tbsp. berries to 8 oz. of boiling water; steep 5 to 10 minutes; strain and drink one cup each morning. This contains the weakest concentration of vitex.

Tincture: Use 40 drops of the 1:5 tincture each morning.

Standardized extract capsules: Use one 175 mg capsule each morning.

Poke root oil or salve rubbed on the breast will help to decrease inflammation and tenderness.

Liver and Lymphatic Tincture

2 parts milk thistle seed
2 parts dandelion root
1 part burdock root
1 part fenugreek seed
1 part cleavers
1 part licorice root

Use ½ to 1 tsp. 3 times a day for several weeks along with vitex and evening primrose oil.

Menopause

Menopause is a natural phase of a woman's menstrual life. At some point, probably around age 40 or so, changes in hormone regulation begin to signal the ultimate cessation of periods. This time when periods are still experienced, though perhaps irregularly, is known as the climacteric and it can go on for many years before periods actually stop. Cessation of periods itself is known as menopause. This usually occurs between 50 and 60 years of age.

Some women experience little or no discomfort during the climacteric and after menopause. Others have a more difficult time with the changes. Symptoms that may be experienced before and after menopause include sleep disturbances, menstrual irregularities, vaginal dryness, emotional ups and downs, temperature intolerance or hot flashes, night sweats, itchiness of the vulva, lowered libido and others. As hormone regulation changes and hormones necessary for reproduction are diminished in their secretion, many changes begin to occur in the body. Some of the symptoms result from those changes.

The views society has about menopause and the aging woman play an important role in a woman's experience of menopause. Aging women are often seen in our society as sexless creatures who have completed their reproductive role and no longer have an important place in society. Women often feel that their very important nurturing role as mother has also been completed, leading them to wonder what use they are to their families, as well. The accompanying emotional considerations with this societal image are enormous and play a major role in determining how a woman experiences the menopausal period. With so much of her identity wrapped up in her reproductive cycle it is no wonder that the prospect of the cessation of that cycle can send a woman onto an emotional rollercoaster.

Some women can take their menopausal changes in stride while others are deeply affected by the severity of their symptoms. Sleep disturbances, temperature intolerance, mood swings and the like make some women's daily lives nearly unbearable. It is then that relief is often sought. In addition, there is the expectation for some women that they will experience a miserable decade or so as they undergo these profound changes. Friends have been through it, horror stories have been told and fear of the unknown begins to develop. Symptom relief may be a necessary pursuit in many of these cases.

Conventional Medical Treatment

As stated earlier, hormones responsible for the continuing cycle of changes in a woman's reproductive system also have their effects on other parts of the body. In recent years much has been said about these effects as they relate to estrogen. Estrogen has been shown to have effects on bone metabolism, vascular health and mental alertness. Interestingly, studies on these physiological changes focus on estrogen for women, while comparable studies in males focus on other factors such as diet and lifestyle. The reasons for this seem confusing. Is it the well-intentioned medical system which seeks to enhance a woman's aging process, or is it just another example of America's love affair with pharmaceutical products and the "quick fix"? Nature has seen fit to discontinue the reproductive process in woman when her children are grown, at an age when life turns inward and aging naturally occurs. For most women, the natural way seems to work just fine without pharmaceutical intervention.

The claims of estrogen's many benefits include prevention of osteoporosis, prevention of heart disease and prevention of senility. Taking hormones to replace those which had been naturally produced in the body may have an effect on these disease processes according to some studies. Women who are at high risk for these diseases may want to discuss the pros and cons of hormone replacement therapy (HRT). However, long-term studies of the side effects of HRT are lacking, and there is some evidence to show that the risk of some cancers is considerably increased with its use. Any woman considering the use of HRT should ask her doctor for information on the risks of such treatment.

Before even considering HRT, the risk factors for these disease processes (other then estrogen "deficiency") should be explored. Family history of osteoporosis and heart disease, for example, should be investigated. A woman's lifestyle including nicotine use, the use of over-the-counter medications and prescription medications should be explored and discussed. Dietary habits should also be reviewed to see whether vitamins and minerals necessary for healthy bone and for a healthy cardiovascular system are being consumed or taken supplementally. Is the diet high in phosphates as are found in sodas and fast foods? This can cause a problem with normal mineral regulation in the body and bone construction. Diets high in saturated fats and in refined carbohydrates (sugars, breads, pasta) will eventually result in high cholesterol and triglyceride values in the blood, known risk factors for heart disease and stroke. Excess caffeine can also deplete minerals necessary for proper bone metabolism. Low stomach acid or poor absorption in the digestive tract might lead to insufficient levels of the vitamins and minerals necessary for bone and cardiovascular as well as brain and central nervous system function.

These factors should all be explored and helpful changes made before the use of HRT is even considered. If a woman chooses to take HRT without correcting these potential imbalances in her physiology, her risk for serious side effects is increased since her body is less able to control and deal with the extra hormonal levels.

Antidepressants are also frequently prescribed to deal with the mood changes sometimes associated with the climacteric and menopause. These powerful drugs have a long list of side effects. Any woman whose doctor has prescribed antidepressants should ask many questions before considering taking them.

Natural and Herbal Treatments

Diet

The diet for menopause is generally geared towards optimizing normal hormonal balance, not by replacing the hormones, but rather by ensuring that the body undergoes its changes with a minimum of discomfort and problems. A diet rich in whole grains, fresh fruits and vegetables, uncontaminated water, low in animal protein and saturated fats is best. Sea vegetables are very helpful in replacing the minerals that seem to be deficient as we age. Eliminating caffeine helps to avoid problems with body temperature regulation. A diet rich in relaxing foods (little meat or sugar or refined carbohydrates) enhances overall well-being during the climacteric and menopause. Unless they are not tolerated well, organic dairy products might help with calcium loss. This is especially important where there is an increased risk for osteoporosis.

Supplements

A balanced formula of vitamins and minerals can be very helpful at this time. In particular vitamin E can soften the symptoms that accompany the menopausal period including hot flushes. Often 800 IU of vitamin E in conjunction with borage seed oil (3,000 mg a day) will be enough to stop the temperature regulation problems. Vitamin E has also proven to be protective against heart disease along with folic acid (which should be in the multivitamin). Additional calcium and magnesium along with boron and vitamin K may be helpful in reducing the risk for osteoporosis by enhancing the body's production of bone matrix.

Herbal Treatments

Herbal treatments for menopause vary depending on the symptoms experienced and their degree of severity. It is a good idea to help the hormonal changes along with the use of vitex for balancing of the pituitary. Additionally, wild yam and soybean creams and oral preparations have been shown to aid in the balance of estrogen and progesterone. Phytoestrogens (see page 75) are good choices as they help in conditions of excess estrogen as well as in cases such as menopause where estrogen decreases considerably.

When nervous tension or insomnia are experienced during menopause, try nervine herbs such as motherwort, skullcap, passionflower, lemonbalm and oatstraw. If anxiety does not reduce with these herbs, kava kava should be considered.

Vaginal Infections

Vaginal infections are among the most common health problems reported by women. Vaginal infections may be caused by several different types of microorganisms, the most common being yeast and bacteria. Yeast infections are often associated with a white curdlike discharge, itching of the labial area and red irritated skin. They may also be accompanied by rectal itching and digestive disturbances. Vaginal yeast infections are often associated with antibiotic use and a diet high in refined sugar, fruit and fruit juices. Bacterial infections have a thin white to gray discharge, odor and little itching or discomfort. Bacteria changes the vaginal pH to alkaline instead of the normal acid pH, so using a white distilled vinegar douche can be helpful in resolving the problem.

Women who are plagued with chronic yeast or bacterial infections and who have not been able to heal themselves successfully may be suffering from more than a yeast infection. With repetitive infection and use of vaginal treatments, the vaginal environment changes, shifting away from the normal microflora and towards a flora in which the yeasts and bacteria start to cause chronic irritation. Many times the microflora shifts significantly and a series of cultures may be necessary to get the correct diagnosis.

We suggest running a Vaginosis Profile from the Great Smokies Laboratory in Asheville, North Carolina (1-800-522-4762). It helps to put the whole vaginal picture together and shows if intestinal microflora are connected to the problem. Other factors which may contribute to chronic vaginal irritation include constipation, poor hygiene, vaginal allergy to a soap, detergent or chemicals and sexual reinfection. All of these possibilities need to be investigated and addressed in the overall treatment in order to break the cycle. The treatments for chronic vaginal infection include reducing the infection, avoiding reinfection, strengthening the immune system, restoring normal vaginal microflora and pH and correcting digestive flora and function.

Conventional Medical Treatments

Conventional medical treatments for chronic vaginosis rely on antibiotic and antifungal creams, douches and suppositories for a strictly topical approach.

Natural and Herbal Treatments

If you suffer from chronic vaginal irritation or infection it is important for you to follow a diet low in sugars and refined carbohydrates. You should eat mostly whole foods, organic vegetables, unsweetened yogurt with live acidophilus cultures, moderate amounts of whole fruit, lots of leafy greens and a minimum of red meat. Support the immune system with tonic herbs like burdock, nettles, red clover, oat straw, astragalus and dandelion. Avoid constipation, use "peri-wash" in a squirt bottle to clean after every stool or urination, avoid bath oils and avoid washing with harsh soaps.

Topical treatments include suppositories, herbal douches, herbal peri-washes, creams and ointments. These should be used regularly 3 to 4 times a day with acute infections and 1 to 2 times a day with chronic infections. Herbal preparations can be made from herbs whose actions are anti-microbial such as echinacea root, myrrh, tea tree, oregano, thyme, goldenseal root and bloodroot; astringent herbs such as witch hazel bark, yarrow flowers, bayberry root bark or white oak bark to strengthen the membranes; demulcent herbs such as calendula flowers, comfrey leaf or root, slippery elm bark or marshmallow root to soothe the irritated skin and the itch. For chronic vaginal irritation use mucous membrane toners such as calendula flowers, comfrey leaf or root, red clover flowers, goldenseal root and plantain leaf.

Herbal Peri-wash

The use of an herbal wash to rinse the perineum or labia and rectal area regularly can be very helpful in reducing the spreading of infectious agents from the rectal area to the vaginal area. Cleanse the affected area with an antiseptic wash and apply some of the wash with a squirt bottle so that the force of the liquid stream dislodges some of the microbes. A simple wash can be made from a strong infusion of oregano, thyme, rosemary or sage leaves. Here are two useful recipes.

Antifungal Peri-wash

Mix the following in a 1-oz amber bottle:

- ¼ oz. tea tree oil
- ¼ oz. yarrow tincture
- ¼ oz. myrrh tincture
- ¼ oz. calendula tincture

Shake well. Add 1 tsp. of the mix to 4 oz. warm water. Put in a squirt bottle and apply as needed.

Antibacterial Peri-wash

Mix the following in a 1-oz amber bottle:

- ¼ oz. goldenseal tincture
- ¼ oz. echinacea tincture
- ¼ oz. myrrh tincture
- ¼ oz. lavender flower tincture

Shake well. Add 1 tsp. of the mix to 4 oz. warm water. Put in a squirt bottle and apply as needed.

Creams and Salves

Herbal creams and salves may be used for irritation of the labia or vulva area. If the area is raw and cracked, use herbal salves to protect the area with their oily cover. If the area is very itchy, hot and burning, use herbal creams to cool and soothe the area. Choose herbs which act as an antiseptic such as echinacea, goldenseal, thuja, tea tree, white sage, lavender flowers or myrrh. Creams and salves should also contain vulnerary herbs to encourage healing of the skin. Herbs which fall into this group include calendula flowers, comfrey root or leaf, chamomile flowers, yarrow flowers, plantain leaf or witch hazel.

Urinary Tract Infections

The most common site for problems with the urinary tract in women is at the bladder or the urethra, given its close proximity to the vagina and rectum. The bladder or urethra might not be infected, but it might be very irritated from exposure to chemicals or frequent intercourse. If there is irritation of the urethra or if there is a feeling of discomfort in the lower abdomen, a urine sample may be helpful in determining the cause of the symptoms. If there are signs in the urine that indicate the possibility of an infection, the sample can be cultured to see what organisms are present in order to determine which treatment to use.

Common signs and symptoms of a UTI include difficulty urinating, pain on urination, urgency, incontinence, frequent urination and discomfort in the lower abdomen. If the infection has traveled up the urinary tract toward the kidney, the patient may experience fever, chills and lower back pain as well.

Conventional Medical Treatments

Generally there is no treatment for irritation of the urethra and the bladder. If there is an infection or a suspicion of one, antibiotics are usually given, especially in the form of sulfa drugs.

Natural and Herbal Treatments

When suffering from a urinary tract infection, first and foremost slow down and rest. Take a little extra time off from your daily routine. Drink lots of fluids during the day to flush the urinary system, about eight ounces of fluid every hour. Alternating between soothing medicated herbal teas, water and unsweetened cranberry juice during the day works well. The cranberry makes the urethra slippery, thereby making it harder for the bacteria to adhere and settle in the area. It must be unsweetened because avoiding natural and refined sugars is important. Cranberry is also available in concentrated gel caps which can be taken easily with water. Use two 250 mg capsules 3 to 4 times a day for acute infections and one time a day to prevent infections if you are particularly prone to them. Avoid the following:

- Caffeine: tea, coffee, chocolate, soft drinks.
- High acid foods: orange juice, tomatoes, too much fruit.
- Vaginal soaps, deodorants, sanitary napkins, noncotton underwear.
- Sexual activity.

We recommend taking the herbs in tea or tincture form rather than in capsules but if only capsules are available, be sure to take them with a full glass of water. Teas and tinctures should be taken three to five times a day if treating an acute infection. Medicinal herbs to include in a urinary formula would include antiseptic herbs such as goldenseal, thyme, juniper berry, garlic, uva ursi and yarrow flowers; soothing demulcent herbs such as marshmallow root, slippery elm bark, cornsilk or calendula flowers; and urinary astringent herbs such as horsetail, parsley, celery seed, couch grass, birch bark and buchu leaves.

Diuretic-acting herbs taken as teas such as dandelion root, cornsilk, celery seed, parsley, horsetail and birch bark encourage flushing of the urinary system.

Herbal Tincture for UTIs

Mix the following tinctures in a 2 oz. bottle:

½ oz. thyme
½ oz. goldenseal
½ oz. uva ursi
¼ oz. echinacea
¼ oz. ginger

Use ½ tsp. in 4 oz. of warm water every 2 hours until symptoms are gone. Continue at two doses a day for several days after the symptoms are gone.

Tea for Cystitis

Mix ½ cup each of the following herbs:

Uva ursi leaves
Cornsilk
Parsley leaf
Thyme leaves
Celery seed
Fennel seed
Cinnamon bark
Lavender flowers

Use 3 Tbsp. of the herb mix to 16 oz. of boiling water; steep 10 minutes, strain and drink ½ cup every hour when acute or 2 to 3 cups daily if mild.

Useful Facts About Herbs

Making Herbal Preparations

Many herbal preparations are easy to make at home. Making your own herbal preparations such as teas, decoctions, oils, salves and extracts can be simple and lots of fun.

Teas (Infusions)

The aerial parts of an herb, such as leaves and flowers and sometimes soft berries and seeds, are used for infusions or teas. The standard proportion is 1 tsp. herb to 1 cup water. Pour the boiling water over the herb, cover, and let stand for 10 to 20 minutes. Most infusions should be used within 8 to 12 hours or can be stored in the refrigerator up to 3 days.

Decoctions

The hard or woody parts of the plant such as the roots, seeds and barks are used for decoctions. The proportions are the same as for an infusion, 1 teaspoon per cup. Place the herb in cold water, bring to a boil, simmer 5 to 20 minutes, remove from heat and strain. Use within 8 to 12 hours or store in the refrigerator for up to 3 days.

Baths

Use a quart of herbal infusion or a decoction depending on the herbs to be used in the recipe. Strain the herbs out and add to the bath.

Compresses

These are for external applications. Make up a quart of an infusion or decoction as described above; use a flannel cloth or washcloth as the compress. Moisten the cloth with the herbal mixture and apply over the affected area; cover with a piece of plastic and a towel to keep the compress warm. Leave on for 15 to 25 minutes.

Poultices

Poultices can be made simply by macerating a fresh herb to a pulp and applying the pulp to the skin. The herb can be macerated by using a mortar and pestle, a blender or by finely chopping it with a knife. Dried herbs can be used if reconstituted with water until moist and soft. Freshly grated roots are easy to make into a poultice. Herbal powder can be used for poultices if mixed with enough warm water to make a paste or gruel. Poultices are placed directly on the area to be healed. They should be applied for 10 to 20 minutes. Cover with cheesecloth topped with plastic wrap to keep heat in.

Tinctures

Tinctures are made by digesting the herb in an alcohol/water mixture for 14 days. They can be made with either fresh or dried herbs and provide a way to preserve the herb's medicinal properties for several years. Officially, the tincture is made by using 1 part herb to 5 parts 100 percent alcohol/water by weight. A simple home method would be to pack a jar with the herb and cover with the alcohol/water solution so that no herb matter is exposed to the air. Let stand for 14 days, press or strain out and pour into amber glass bottles. One hundred percent grain alcohol is the best to use, but a good quality vodka also works. If using vodka, use a 100 proof (50% alcohol) and no dilution with water will be necessary. If using 100 percent grain alcohol, dilute to desired strength, 50 percent alcohol with 50 percent water extracts most active constituents from common medicinal herbs.

Storing Herbs

Pay special attention to how you store your herbs. If they are stored properly, they will last and retain their actions better. Here are a few helpful hints.

Air facilitates oxidation, so fill your containers to the top with the herb or fill the excess space with cotton. Light causes photo-oxidation and accelerates chemical changes in the herb. Thus it is important to use opaque glass storage containers. Temperature also affects the rate of chemical reaction in the plant material. The higher the temperature, the higher the rate of chemical reaction. Ideal storage temperature is 55-65 degrees F. Remove all insects, fungal material, bacteria and other contaminants before putting herbs in storage containers. Airtight containers are best. Try to avoid plastic as it can be broken down by some of the active constituents in herbs. Hard plastic containers are okay for short-term use, but glass is best.

Make sure to protect the herb matter from light by using amber jars or by keeping clear glass jars in an herb closet to shut out the light.

The atmosphere should be dry. All containers should be heated slightly to eliminate condensation, then cooled, and the herb matter put inside immediately. If there is any extra moisture in the jar, the herb will mold. Enzymes stay active in the plant matter at 8 to 10 percent moisture content and cause deterioration.

Most leaves and flowers can be kept up to a year and replenished with a new harvest each growing season. Roots, barks and seeds will store longer as they consist of harder plant materials. They should keep 18 to 36 months.

Appendices

Phytoestrogens: What are They All About?

Phytoestrogens are plant constituents which possess estrogenic activity either by mimicking the action of estrogen in the body or affecting the body's estrogen metabolism. They are generally considered to be weaker than human hormones. Phytoestrogen compounds also vary greatly in their strength and effects on the body. Many plant compounds with phytoestrogenic activity affect the body by acting on the estrogen receptors found in the breast, ovaries and uterus.

The regular use of foods and herbal teas high in phytoestrogens can be helpful in the prevention of reproductive illness as well as in the treatment of many female reproductive diseases. Listed below are some of the conditions where phytoestrogens might help:

- Prevention and treatment of breast cancer and osteoporosis.
- Menopausal and postmenopausal complaints associated with lowered estrogen such as hot flashes, insomnia, anxiety, vaginal dryness.
- Infertility.
- Menstrual irregularities.
- Hyperestrogenic conditions such as ovarian cysts, fibroids, fibrocystic breasts, endometriosis.

Dietary Sources of Phytoestrogens

- Soy contains several different constituents with phytoestrogenic activity. The Japanese diet is high in soy which may be one of the reasons why Japanese women have fewer hormone-dependent cancers, less osteoporosis and less risk of heart disease. Sprouted soy beans have the highest phytoestrogen content. Other forms include soy flour, soy beans, soy flakes, soy milk, tofu, tempeh and miso.
- Legumes: Peas, beans, mung beans, chickpeas.
- Sprouts: Alfalfa, clover, mung, wheat, rye, radish.
- Grains which are whole and unprocessed.
- Cabbage.
- Parsley, seaweeds, celery, carrots, anise, fennel and licorice.
- Olives and olive oil.
- Flaxseeds and other seeds.

Herbs Containing Phytoestrogens

Black Cohosh *(Cimicifuga racemosa)* contains phytoestrogen-acting lignins and isoflavones. It is thought to decrease luteinizing hormone (LH) secretion from the pituitary gland and suppress LH release, making it useful in hot flashes and flushing. Black cohosh is often used with lady's mantle in the treatment of hot flashes and flushing. Combine equal amounts of each tincture and use ½ to 1 tsp. of the mix 3 times a day. This herb has an antispasmodic action on the uterus and pelvic areas, making it useful for menstrual cramps and endometriosis pain. Use 1 to 2 cups decoction per dose or ½ to 1 tsp. of tincture.

Dong Quai *(Angelica sinensis)* has phytoestrogenic

activity and has been shown to compete for receptor sites to block receptor sites thus lowering high estrogen levels, as well as to fill receptor sites to increase low levels of estrogen. Thus we can see that this herb regulates estrogen levels in the body in many ways and thus is useful in the treatment of perimenopausal and menopausal complaints such as hot flashes, irregular bleeding, insomnia or vaginal dryness. Dong quai is also useful in the treatment of menstrual irregularities, PMS, infertility, ovarian cysts and breast cysts. It may be used as a tea (1 cup 3 times a day), tincture (½ tsp. 3 times a day), or in capsules as directed on the bottle.

Licorice *(Glycyrrhiza glabra),* **alfalfa** *(Medicago sativa)* and **red clover** *(Trifolium pratenses)* all contain phytoestrogen-acting isoflavones which act to influence estrogen metabolism, decrease the risk of hormone-dependent cancers, mimic estrogen effects and stimulate breast milk production. These plants all belong to the pea family (the same as soy), all members of which are useful for their phytoestrogen activity. These plants may be used in the treatment of perimenopausal and menopausal symptoms, premenstrual syndrome, menstrual cramps, infertility, polycystic ovaries and fibrocystic breast disease. These herbs may be taken as a tea (one cup 3 times daily), a tincture (½ to 1 tsp. 2 to 3 times a day) or a capsule as directed on the bottle.

The Anti-Estrogenic Diet

1. Eliminate sugar, white flour and refined foods.
2. Eliminate methylxanthines such as coffee, tea,

chocolate, colas and other foods or beverages that contain caffeine.

3. Eliminate red meat and fowl. Organically raised fowl is acceptable in moderate amounts.
4. Decrease fats, especially animal fats, margarine and saturated fats. Instead use unsaturated fats such as those in cold-pressed vegetable oils. Avoid hidden hydrogenated fats in processed or refined foods. These oils are harmful to the body.
5. Decrease foods found in the cabbage family such as broccoli, Brussels sprouts, cauliflower, etc. These foods lower thyroid activity thus disrupting the reproductive cycle.
6. Decrease all dairy products such as milk, cheese, ice cream.
7. Increase complex carbohydrates such as vegetables and whole grains.
8. Increase the consumption of garlic and onions.
9. Be sure that you are taking adequate amounts of selenium, iodine, beta-carotene and vitamins A, C, and E.

Coupling this diet with an adequate intake of fluids and exercise will increase overall good health.

Antiestrogenic Smoothie

Mix the following in a blender:

1 Tbsp. flaxseed oil
½ to 1 tsp. kelp
1 to 2 Tbsp. of granulated lecithin
1 to 2 Tbsp. brewer's yeast
1 Tbsp. chlorella or spirulina
2 organic eggs (optional)
Banana or other fruit

Yogurt or soy yogurt
Drink for breakfast or whenever desired.

Other Helpful Procedures

Castor Oil Packs

Castor oil is an anti-inflammatory agent and has analgesic properties. It can be used for many situations: liver cleansing, inflammation and/or infection (not for open wounds), breast infection and/or plugged milk duct, peptic ulcers, colitis, pelvic problems, arthritis or chest colds.

Equipment needed: flannel or wool cloth, hot water bottle or heating pad, plastic wrap, 4 to 6 ounces of castor oil.

Procedure:

1. Fold a 2 to 4-inch thickness of flannel cloth about 10" × 12" for abdominal applications.
2. Dampen the cloth and pour 4 to 6 oz. of castor oil onto the cloth.
3. Heat castor oil pack in oven on cookie sheet at a low temperature for 20–30 minutes until hot.
4. Place over the treatment area and then put plastic wrap over the castor oil pack.
5. Place heating pad or hot water bottle on top. Pack may remain in place for 1 to 8 hours. Minimal treatment time is one hour. In an acute situation the castor oil pack is used 1 to 3 times

a day. For a more chronic condition, the pack is usually applied 1 to 3 times a week.

6. Clean the castor oil off your body with soda water 1 tsp. baking soda mixed in 1 pint of cool water.
7. Castor oil packs may be kept up to one year in a plastic container or zip lock bag. Store in the refrigerator.

Hot and Cold Alternating Sitz Baths

Sitz baths are useful for increasing circulation to the pelvic area of the body, helping to eliminate a situation in which normal passage of nutrients and wastes has been disrupted by a congestive process. In this way, pain can be alleviated and infections and inflammations can be more readily dealt with by the body.

A sitz bath is a bath which is just deep enough to cover the pelvic area. This means using a tub big enough to put just the buttocks in or filling the bathtub so that the water comes up to one's hip bones. Two tubs are needed as one is filled with hot water and one with cool to cold water. The bathtub and a laundry or dish tub work well.

Start with 5 minutes in the hot tub, then 2 minutes in the cold tub. Repeat the entire process 3 times, ending with the cold tub. Do not submerge the entire body.

FLAXSEED OIL RECIPES

Tips about flaxseed oil:

1. It should always be kept in the refrigerator in a dark bottle to maintain freshness.

2. Never cook with flaxseed oil or heat it on the stove or in the microwave. This destroys the benefits of the oil.
3. The stronger smelling or tasting the flax oil, the less fresh it probably is and should be discarded. Always check the expiration date on the bottle.

Fruit Smoothie

½ banana
2 ice cubes
1 cup juice (apple, pineapple, grape)
1 Tbsp. yogurt
1 Tbsp. flaxseed oil

Add all ingredients together in a blender and mix. Also add protein powder, fresh or frozen berries, cherries or whatever fruit you like. Great for breakfast.

Ginger Dressing

3 Tbsp. flaxseed oil
1 to 2 Tbsp. fresh lemon juice
1 tsp. fresh grated ginger
1 clove garlic, minced

Whisk ingredients together and store in the refrigerator in a dark bottle. Great as a light dressing over salad greens, grains or vegetables.

Tamari Dressing

¼ cup flaxseed oil
2 to 3 Tbsp. tamari
2 to 3 Tbsp. apple cider vinegar
1 to 3 cloves garlic, minced

Adjust these proportions to taste. Whisk ingredients together and store in the refrigerator in a dark bottle. Especially good over grain and/or bean salads.

Glossary of Herbs

COMMON NAME, BOTANICAL NAME AND PART USED

Alfalfa	*Medicago sativa*	Leaf
Anise	*Pimpinella anisum*	Seed
Artichoke	*Cynara scolymus*	Leaf
Astragalus	*Astragalus membranaceus*	Root
Bayberry	*Myrica cerifera*	Rootbark
Birch	*Betula pendula*	Bark
Black cohosh	*Cimicifuga racemosa*	Root
Black haw	*Viburnum prunifolium*	Root, bark
Bloodroot	*Sanguinaria canadensis*	Root
Blue cohosh	*Caulophyllum thalictroides*	Root
Blue vervain	*Verbena hastata*	Root, herb
Buchu	*Agothosma betulina*	leaf
Burdock	*Arctium lappa*	Root
Calendula	*Calendula officinalis*	Flowers
Catnip	*Nepta cateria*	Leaf
Celandine	*Chelidonium majus*	Leaf, flower
Chamomile	*Matricaria recutita*	Flower
Chaparral	*Larrea spp.*	Leaf
Chaste tree	*Vitex agnus-castus*	Berry
Cinnamon	*Cinnamomum spp.*	Bark
Cleavers	*Galium aparine*	Whole herb
Comfrey	*Symphytum officinale*	Root, leaf
Cornsilk	*Zea mays*	Silk
Couch grass	*Agrophyron repens*	Rhizome
Crampbark	*Viburnum opulus*	Bark
Dandelion	*Taraxacum officinalis*	Root, leaf

Dong quai	*Angelica sinensis*	Root
Echinacea	*Echinacea spp.*	Root, leaf
False unicorn	*Helonias lutium*	Root
Fennel	*Foeniculum vulgare*	Seed
Fenugreek	*Trigonella foenum-graecum*	Seed
Garlic	*Allium sativa*	Bulb
Geranium, cranesbill	*Geranium muculatum*	Root
Ginger	*Zingiber officinalis*	Root
Goldenseal	*Hydrastis canadensis*	Root
Horsetail	*Equisetum arvense*	Leaf
Jamaican dogwood	*Piscidia erythrina*	Bark
Juniper	*Juniperus communis*	Berry
Kava kava	*Piper methysticum*	Rhizome
Lady's mantle	*Alchemilla vulgaris*	Leaf
Lavender	*Lavandula spp.*	Flowers
Lemonbalm	*Melissa officinalis*	Leaf
Licorice	*Glycyrrhiza spp.*	Root
Marshmallow	*Althea officinalis*	Root
Milk thistle	*Silybum marianum*	Seed
Motherwort	*Leonurus cardiaca*	Leaf
Myrrh	*Commiphora spp.*	Resin
Nettles	*Urtica dioica*	Leaf
Oatgrass, oatstraw	*Avena sativa*	Stem, leaf
Oregano	*Origanum spp.*	Leaf
Parsley	*Petroselinum crispum*	Leaf
Pasqueflower	*Anemone pulsatilla*	Flower, stem
Passionflower	*Passiflora incarnata*	Whole herb
Plantain	*Plantago spp.*	Whole herb
Prickly ash	*Zanthoxylum spp.*	Bark
Raspberry	*Rubus idaeus*	Leaf

Red clover	*Trifolium pratense*	Flower
Rosemary	*Rosmarinus officinalis*	Leaf
Sage	*Salvia officinalis*	Leaf
Shepherd's purse	*Capsella bursa-pastoris*	Leaf
Skullcap	*Scutellaria spp.*	Whole herb
Slippery elm	*Ulmus fulva*	Inner bark
Squaw vine	*Mitchella repens*	Whole herb
Tea tree	*Melaleuca alternifolia*	Essential oil
Thuja	*Thuja occidentalis*	Leaf
Thyme	*Thymus officinalis*	Whole herb
Turmeric	*Curcuma longa*	Rhizome
Uva ursi	*Arctostephylas uva-ursi*	Leaf
Valerian	*Valeriana officinalis*	Root
White oak	*Quercus alba*	Bark
Wild yam	*Dioscorea villosa*	Root
Witch hazel	*Hamamelis virginiana*	Bark
Yarrow	*Achillea millefolium*	Leaf, flower

Herbal Suppliers

Also contact your local health food/natural food stores as a resource for herbal products.

Avena Botanicals
219 Mill Street
Rockport, ME 04856
(207) 594-0694

Blessed Herbs
109 Barre Plains Road
Oakham, MA 01068
(800) 489-4372

Herbalist and Alchemist
P.O. Box 553
Broadway, NJ 08808
(908) 689-9092

Herb Pharm
P.O. Box 116
Williams, OR 97544
(800) 348-4372

Bibliography

Aldercreutz, Honjo, Higashi et al. Urinary excretion of lignans and bean isoflavonoid phytoestrogens in Japanese men and women consuming a traditional Japanese diet. *Am. J Clin Nutr* 6(1991) 1091–1093.

Berkow, Robert MD, ed. *The Merck Manual of Diagnosis and Therapy.* 16th edition. Rahway, N.J.: Merck Research Laboratories, 1992.

Bisset, Norman Grainger. *Herbal Drugs and Phytopharmaceuticals.* Stuttgart: Medpharm Scientific Publishers, 1994.

British Herbal Medicine Association. *British Herbal Pharmacopoeia.* W. Yorks, England: The British Herbal Medicine Assoc.: 1983.

British Herbal Medicine Association. *British Herbal Compendium.* Vol. 1. Dorset, England: The British Herbal Medicine Assoc., 1992.

Brown, Donald J. *Herbal Prescriptions for Better Health.* Rocklin, Calif.: Prima Publishing, 1996.

Cook, Wm. *Physio-Medical Dispensatory.* Cincinnati, Ohio, 1869. Portland, Or.: Eclectic Medical Publications, 1985.

Crayhon, Robert. *Robert Crayhon's Nutrition Made Simple.* New York: M. Evans and Company Inc., 1994.

Hoffmann, David. Phytoestrogens, receptors, and the

phytotherapist. *The Protocol Journal of Botanical Medicine,* Vol 1, #4 pp. 8–10. 1996.

Holt, Stephen MD. *Soya for Health.* Larchmont, N.Y.: Mary Ann Liebert Inc., 1996.

Krause and Mahan. *Food, Nutrition and Diet Therapy,* 7th edition. Philadelphia, Pa.: W.B. Saunders Co., 1984.

Kennedy, A.R. The evidence for soybean products as cancer preventive agents. *J Nutr* 123 (3 Suppl) 1995.

McIntyre, Anne. *The Complete Woman's Herbal.* New York: Henry Holt and Company, 1994

Murray, M., and Pizzorno, J. *Encyclopedia of Natural Medicine.* Rocklin, Calif.: Prima Publishing, 1990.

Snow, Joanne Marie. *The Protocol Journal of Botanical Medicine,* Vol 1, #4 pp. 17–23. 1996

Weiss, Rudolf Fritz. *Herbal Medicine.* Translated from the 6th edition by A.R. Meuss. Beaconsfield, England: Beaconfield Publishers, 1988.

INDEX